12 lbs.
of Fudge

12 lbs. of Fudge

WEIGHT LOSS AND MANAGEMENT

AS NATURE INTENDED

Vanessa Victor-Linkenhoker, MD

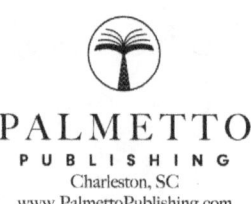

PALMETTO
PUBLISHING
Charleston, SC
www.PalmettoPublishing.com

Copyright © 2023 by Vanessa Victor-Linkenhoker, MD

All rights reserved

No portion of this book may be reproduced, stored in a retrieval system, or transmitted in any form by any means–electronic, mechanical, photocopy, recording, or other–except for brief quotations in printed reviews, without prior permission of the author.

Paperback ISBN: 979-8-8229-3117-6

Dedication

To David and Anna who had to share their mother with thousands of kids over the years. For the missed awards ceremonies, field trips, assemblies, and sporting events. Love, mom.

Synopsis

This is the definitive book on weight loss and management. Even medical terminology is explained and illustrated so simply that a child can follow and apply the concepts. It is an engaging, step by step, instructional manual toward a natural, no gimmick way to manage weight and a healthy lifestyle. There are no pills or injections involved and therefore no side effects. You can "eat the cheesecake" and "eat the bread". Determination and effort are all that's required to implement this life-changing journey.

This instruction is applicable for individuals, but also suitable for group programs, and as an aid to medical professionals and weight management coaches.

Contents

Foreword ix
Chapter 1   Eat to Live 1
Chapter 2   Habits and the Satiety Center 5
Chapter 3   Fuel Up vs Mindless Eating 9
Chapter 4   The Cut/How to—Portion Sizes 13
Chapter 5   12 lbs. of Fudge/Doggy Bag It 18
Chapter 6   Sweat Equity 23
Chapter 7   Accountability 27
Chapter 8   Medical Concepts Made Simple. 30
Chapter 9   Medical Concepts Made Simple. 35
Chapter 10   New Habits and Recap 39

Foreword

Having been at the frontlines of the growing overweight and obesity epidemic for over 20 years as a physician, counseling on weight reduction has become a daily part of the advice I dispense. Type 2 Diabetes is no longer referred to as Adult-Onset Diabetes as it has become increasingly present in adolescents and children.

While it is easy to point fingers at the sheer prevalence of food, for example, in fast food restaurants, school meal programs, and the abundance of food advertising, most food consumption occurs at home and/or associated with family activities. There is a societal tendency towards overindulgence.

There needs to be a fundamental shift in the mindset and approach to food, both individually and within households. New habits need to be established so food is viewed with a "take it or leave it" attitude with less compulsion to overindulge.

Fad diet programs are not a solution, as they are not sustainable. "Eat to live, don't live to eat," is a cliché that I learned from my grandmother and that phrase embodies my approach to weight management. This approach is presented in the manner in which I dispense advice in my practice day to day. Complex medical concepts are explained simply. It is a sound, natural way to halt the progressive accumulation of weight and gradually lose weight while establishing habits and lifestyle changes that can last a lifetime. I have collected clichés, proverbs, and pithy sayings as a hobby and felt a need to share some at the beginning of each chapter.

I hope the sayings here complement the information imparted and I endeavor to drive home a simple, natural, weight loss approach that is engaging and has the feeling of a personal motivational conversation.

"Eat to live, don't live to eat."

CHAPTER 1

Eat to Live

The "Eat to Live" approach to weight management will lead you to acquire a new mindset on eating and weight management. Quit the dietary gimmicks, serial starvation and deprivation and live a little, eat some bread and cheesecake while you lose weight, maintain a healthy weight, and establish habits that can last a lifetime. Eating can be savored, and is an integral part of our celebrations, social interactions, and even business. Why not at these functions enjoy a good steak with the sides, a mouthwatering lasagna with garlic bread, and a delectable dessert. Who doesn't look forward to a Thanksgiving meal, except if you're the one having to prepare the turkey and most of the trimmings; not to mention cleaning up and handwashing the fine China? Have some fixings with your turkey and leave room for desserts. If Aunt Lizzy's casserole is notorious for not being up to scratch, you still have the excuse that you're on a weight reduction program to pass on it. However, if it's the legendary casserole that is to die for, have a serving without guilt. (However), if you eat once a week like it's Thanksgiving, there's a price to pay. Everything in moderation is fine. It's excess that "hurts you". That's even true for fame and fortune, just look around a bit. Regardless of how you look at food, for example, as a delight, indulgence, or therapy; in the long run, it basically boils down to how we're designed to obtain fuel and sustenance. To be deprived of sufficient sustenance results in malnutrition, possibly starvation, and their consequences. Overindulging leads to levels of overweight and obesity with culminative consequences. It is no different for babies and children as it is for adolescents, and adults. In over 20 years of medical practice, I've seen the march toward abnormal weight gain seeming to begin at about 8 to 10 years of age and accelerate from there, sometimes, quite rapidly. However, it can begin and accelerate at any age and often during adolescence and adulthood. My simple principle for weight management is: Intake vs. what you burn over time.

$$\text{Intake} = \text{burn} \rightarrow \text{maintain weight}$$
$$\text{Intake} < \text{burn} \rightarrow \text{lose weight}$$
$$\text{Intake} > \text{burn} \rightarrow \text{gain weight}$$

If you are an elite athlete like an Olympic grade swimmer, you can easily eat more than 3000 calories per meal. When you retire from training and competing at that level, you must cut back on your caloric intake. On the other hand, if you are an elite athlete who does not consume enough calories, you'd lose weight, have hormonal and organ disturbances eventually and fail to keep up with training at that level. There is an actual diagnosis of "Failure to Thrive" which is encountered most often in neonates and the elderly but may occur at any time when the caloric intake is not sufficient for growth or maintenance of a healthy weight. In these instances, the investigation centers on whether there is just insufficient intake or underlying illness causing lack of utilization of intake.

To resolve an issue, the most effective and efficient method is to find the root cause and apply the solution there. For too many issues in life as in society, the approach is to spend lots of time and money trying to affect the peripheral issues or the end products while skirting the root cause so that the problem is never resolved. It is akin to being on an endless roller coaster with no progress but always more dips and spins. Weight management is one such issue. We are constantly bombarded with lots of products and programs for weight loss that do not address the root cause and they cannot create a sustainable mindset and lifestyle for healthy weight management.

While examples abound of missing the root cause to solve an issue, to illustrate, imagine that you begin to wake up with back or hip pain that is becoming persistent, but worse upon waking up. You contemplate seeing a chiropractor or orthopedic physician. There could be manipulations, massages, medications (pills, injections), x-rays, MRI's, physical therapy, and a host of interventions that may be applied to this problem, with varying degrees of temporary relief. You might have saved considerable expenditure of time and money if you'd figured out that the pain being worse upon waking up may be related to your sleep position and your mattress. You turn the mattress over and get relief without medicine or medical interventions. There may be need in the future for additional mattress turnings, or eventually procuring a new mattress, or foam pad or body pillow based on your budget, but this is the most efficient solution as the root cause is a one position side sleeper, who is getting older, with a less flexible skeleton and a worn pattern in the mattress. While some may identify with this very scenario, others may have different experiences with different root causes. The point is that one might spend a lot of time and money attending to the symptom while missing the basic solution, for not figuring out the root of the problem. Root cause analysis and applying the solution to the cause is the most beneficial approach to a matter.

It's your level of consumption compared to your level of activity that determines your body habitus over time. So, when I'm told, "Johnny doesn't eat much," while he is crossing percentile lines on a growth chart, my response is that the weight gain is revealing that Johnny is consistently eating more than he is burning for his level of activity. You can basically eat the foods that you like and lose or maintain your weight. Have some cheesecake, have some bread (it's a staple throughout the world), and enjoy a dinner party or business lunch as much as the next person. It's the persistent excess that gets you in trouble. Discard the pills and supplements offered for weight loss. All medications and supplements have the potential for undesirable side effects, even over-the-counter medications, and supplements. And because it's labeled "natural" doesn't mean it can't harm you or that it's good for you. Quit the ever-evolving fad diets and miracle weight loss programs unless you desire a quick round on the endless roller coaster of weight loss and weight gain.

The mindset of looking at food differently and developing a healthy approach to eating can be implemented at any age and will be explained in this book. This program can be employed individually, as a parent to a child, or in a group/support setting. It only requires adopting this approach and the determination to make long-term changes to eating and lifestyle habits.

Eat to live, enjoy occasions as they arrive to break bread in varied settings. Healthy eating habits will serve for a lifetime. Break the dieting fads.

"Train up a child in the way he/she should go." —Prov 22:6
"Old habits die hard."

CHAPTER 2

Habits and the Satiety Center

After infancy, we settle into a pattern of eating 3 meals per day with one or two snacks. If you habitually eat three meals a day, and get busy enough, you will tend to miss one or both snacks, which isn't a bad thing for most of us from time to time. Where food is plentiful, it is easy to overindulge without any realization. Once habits are formed, it takes major lifestyle adjustments to reverse the course. We are after all creatures of habit. It is said that it takes about three weeks of consistent work to change a habit.

Eating, along with weight loss and maintenance should not be hard work though. You do not need to starve yourself, deprive yourself of your favorite foods, count calories i.e., making a math class of every meal, or make a reading class of it by reading and studying labels ad nauseum. If you have allergies to foods and additives, you do need to pay attention to the ingredients in food- there are exceptions to rules.

It is fashionable today to shift the blame for being overweight and the obesity epidemic to fast food restaurants, eating out, school lunch, teachers rewarding kids with snacks, advertising, and a myriad of other scapegoats. However, most of the excess caloric intake is occurring in the home or in family unit settings. I contend therefore, that we'd have to close the supermarkets, whole food stores, as well as the usual scapegoats like fast food and school lunch, which are blamed for the population's ever-increasing girth, if we do not approach this issue honestly.

We've all heard of people who have set out to and have proven that one may eat three meals per day at a fast-food restaurant for three to four months and lose weight. We've also heard the joke about the person who orders a double or triple patty burger loaded with everything, super-sized French fries, an apple pie and Danish, and a diet soda. At this, we all jest "yeah, like that diet soda will really seal the deal on that order". The pearl here is that it is the portion sizes that primarily need to be adjusted. Along with that, the habit of eating or drinking calories constantly throughout the day is the other major contributor, as even drinking sweetened beverages all day can add a significant number of calories to one's diet without awareness.

At the birth of the fast-food industry, the initial burgers were equivalent to the burgers in the current kid's meal. One can still get that portion today by ordering a small burger with a small fry and a small drink, even without ordering a kid's meal in some instances. I still get a kid's meal when I go through a drive-through for lunch and can make it to dinner. Portion sizes have increased to the extent that you give an average ten-year-old a kiddy meal and they'd probably look at you with crossed eyes, wanting to know if that's their full meal.

Habits for the necessary lifestyle changes to acquire include some of the following.

Do get in three meals per day. Three fueling stops per day should sustain us through most human endeavors.

Do make the portion sizes reasonable and sustaining, especially the snack portions. If the snacks are loaded portions and you get 2 or more snacks regularly, you've repeatedly violated the three meal per day habit and consumed the equivalent of five to six meals per day. It should be clear now how snacks can defeat the effort of weight management. Keep snacks to one handful instead of a bag, one or two scoops in a small bowl instead of a heaping bowl full. The handful rule applies to kids as well, their handful instead of an adult's handful.

Habits are more easily formed than broken. Start forming profitable habits early that can serve for a lifetime. If you're a parent whose child is climbing the weight chart compared to the height chart at their well visits, you need to help that child develop the habit of 3 reasonable meals a day and limited snacks. You may even have to use psychology with little children so that one child gets a pudding snack while the other gets a plain flavored gelatin snack at the same sitting, as one needs to gain weight while the other needs to lose or stop gaining weight. Be mindful that similar portion sizes may have vastly different numbers of calories. The caloric density in the example above does not even require calculation as to the objective of consuming a snack with limited vs increased calories. Those decisions can be very intuitive. If you're a teenager or adult who is needing to constantly increase your pant waist size or dress size, stop, change your current "eating habits" to three reasonable meals per day and limited snacks. Your need is to provide enough fuel and you can eat what you like and what you normally eat to a large extent, but you should not repeatedly overeat. It's actually fine to feel a bit peckish by the time you're due to eat your next meal. It's probably a good thing.

Don't skip meals believing that you're helping yourself to not gain weight. I've observed that most of the teenagers and young adults whom I've counseled regarding weight reduction are skipping one or two meals per day, especially breakfast, while steadily gaining too much weight. At some point, either by snacking or consuming larger portions later in the day, they are more than making up for the missed meals. Additionally, my theory on why people skip one or two meals a day and continue to gain weight is as follows. The brain senses the lack of one or two meals and perceives an impending famine or significant deprivation. A part of the survival instinct is to preserve the remaining intake and store reserves for the possible further deprivation that is likely coming. That is, the body becomes more efficient in turning calories into storage so that one may survive a few weeks to months of starvation if the need arises. In the abundance of food, that famine is not about to happen, but the storage substrate of the body is fat. Adipose tissue is being deposited as increased weight/girth, fatty liver, and the result of the skipped meals is counterproductive to the intended purpose.

Don't snack regularly at bedtime or late at night, just because you usually stay up late. You won't burn off any of that snack and will be wearing it plain and simple. If you're at a party, fete, late night hangout, movie, or other get together, then by all means, we all indulge from time to time. Make a "habit" of it and you're toast, pardon the pun.

Don't participate in serial crash diets. Although humanly speaking, there may be a rare need to lose weight quickly to fit into a wedding or bridesmaid dress for example, the roller coaster win-lose cycle is self-defeating and more demoralizing than it is worth.

The satiety center, which is the part of your being that says you're full or satisfied concerning food, is not in your belly, but rather in your brain. If you play faddish brain games with dieting and starving, you set up poor signals between your brain and target organs, referred to as biofeedback. This causes bad biochemistry and psychology and a self-defeating biofeedback loop that makes it impossible to be successful at weight loss and management. It then doesn't matter how many diets and exercise programs you try. The battle is lost before it ensues. I will elaborate on this later, particularly in addressing "Insulin Resistance."

"Too swift arrives as tardy as too slow."
—Shakespeare

CHAPTER 3

Fuel Up vs Mindless Eating

Think of food as fuel, or gas for your car. In the final analysis, the main reason for food is to provide energy to keep you going, although it can provide delectable pleasures.

You can't fill the gas tank of your car every ten or twenty miles down the road or highway. It is not necessary, it would be too much work, and it is just not feasible. Also, the gas tank is not expandable to accommodate over filling. A fair amount of the fuel needs to be burned off before it is reasonable to refuel, even though the gas price is an attractive twenty cents less per gallon ten miles down the road. There may be instances where it's advantageous to refuel because the price is great compared to what you expect to pay on other portions on a journey, but you may only put in a limited number of gallons if the tank is not empty.

There is also no need to refuel your body 10–20 minutes after a meal. Unfortunately, your body will accept the refueling unlike your car's gas tank but will have to store it somewhere. That somewhere may be your liver, waistline, hips, and other undesirable places. Get the picture, while lounging and not engaged in physical exercise, i.e., watching TV, playing videogames, scrolling through social media, or even mostly sitting all day on your job, on a molecular level you're probably not active enough to require refueling in 10–20-minute intervals. Like a parked car in neutral, your body uses a minimal amount of energy while you're inactive, to keep basic functions and organs running, but you're not burning up much fuel (many calories). It would require longer time intervals or less fuel to fill it back to capacity. Eating from boredom or just because food/snacks are available is mindless, inappropriate and the major cause of many of the problems with excess weight gain and obesity.

I am often told of kids whining about being hungry 10–20 minutes after having eaten a full meal. They require snack food then and this process is replicated on a regular basis. Teens and adults act similarly, except for the ability to procure their own snacks. One can't be "truly" hungry shortly after having a full meal, just as your car can't require refueling after burning up a couple of gallons of gas. It is inconceivable, but is a reality for many people—do you identify with this scenario? What's happened here for a child or adult who truly feels hungry shortly after a meal, is that the biofeedback loop for satiety (feeling satisfied after a meal) is disrupted. Your brain is receiving bad signals. Poor eating habits over a long period of time have resulted in disrupted biochemistry and a state of Insulin Resistance is now one of your biggest hindrances to getting the weight back under control. I will elaborate on this concept later in chapter 8 and provide advice on how to overcome this obstacle.

Constant grazing, overeating, coupled with relative inactivity can cause significant as well as rapid weight gain. I have seen kids put on twenty to thirty pounds over the course of a summer vacation. When the eating habits are not addressed and the process continues unabated, the results can be very difficult to reverse. In some cases, the child's weight quickly expands so that the weight may have to be plotted on the growth chart well above the allotted area of a weight chart and occasionally into the portion above that is allotted for the height chart. In this case, the child goes from slender to obese in a couple of years and may proceed to becoming morbidly obese. Those habits are hard to break once established, and significant weight gain is not as easily lost as gained. Again, if your car is parked for an extended period of time, you do not use up gas unless something is fundamentally wrong like a leak, or the fuel has been siphoned off. For the less active, sedentary person who does no sports, very little walking, or other exercise, you need less fuel. If you are a high-powered athlete, you may need to consume up to 3–4 thousand calories per meal at your peak, conditioning and competing. Fuel consumption, i.e., caloric intake, must be reduced when you stop training and being very active. Fueling up must match the requirement for equilibrium, growth, and weight reduction, as the case may be.

Let's say you are the kind of person or family who comes out of one store at a shopping center and gets into your vehicle, drive, and park in front of another store in the same plaza to shop, perhaps you do not need the meal sized snack during that shopping spree when a smaller snack will fit the bill. Then to top off the shopping experience, not too long after the meal sized snack, you pull up to a restaurant to have a complete meal with appetizer, bread, entrée, and dessert consuming every morsel. Since you ate out early, and are staying up late, there's a late-night snack in the picture as well. All of this occurred after lunch in addition to what was consumed up to lunch time and any grazing opportunities also taken advantage of. This is a very familiar tableau, but it illustrates the ease with which excessive fuel stops can occur in a day. Let's keep the fuel stops and remove the shopping, so that we did not even engage in the short walks between the car and the stores as we drove from one store to another, and the caloric consumption becomes even more excessive.

Additionally, I may like a particular flavor of soda, ice cream, or pastry, and not feel compelled to consume it every day. Have it as a treat occasionally, savor the taste and recall "why I love this dish or desert". The habitual, almost ritual, and excessive consumption is what is detrimental to too many.

Be the master of your consumption of food and not the slave. Have a "taste", resist the "binge". Resist the indulgence just because it's available and especially because of boredom. Fuel up to match activity levels and energy needs.

Recall that persistent weight gain occurs because of consistently taking in a lot more calories than you burn. The greater the imbalance between intake and burning, the more persistent and evolving the problem. That's why all diet programs must restrict your caloric intake in one way or another. Many try to manipulate caloric intake by unnatural means though, like restricting certain categories of foods and trying to trick your body into burning off stored calories. Some even lead you to accept that the diarrhea and excess ketones are just a part of the price to pay. However, the stress on your organs comes with consequences and eliminating entire categories of foods is not sustainable over long periods of time and certainly not for a lifetime. It's also not a pleasurable way of eating. Remember eating can also be varied and pleasurable and there's a world of food out there waiting to be sampled.

"A thousand-mile journey begins with one step."

CHAPTER 4

The Cut/How to—Portion Sizes

So, you've decided that the best course of action is to institute a healthy lifestyle change of eating three reasonable meals per day with one or 2 snacks. Here comes the "cut" and please read on, because it is not at all painful or faddish. It's quite elementary.

Your goal for weight loss, regardless of the weight that you're starting from should be reasonable, achievable, and geared for success. It must be in increments that can be replicated so that the same habits formed for the initial weight reduction can be reinforced as goals are attained and reset.

"The Tithe—10%"
I propose to think of it as a tithe, or an investment type of pay yourself first percentage. My advice is to aim to lose 10% of your current weight in three to six months regardless of the starting weight. Once that goal is achieved, reset for the next 10%. I am often asked "what should be my ideal weight?" My response is that we're not working toward an ideal weight at this point, but to lose 10% of your current weight. From where some are starting, looking at ideal weight would be discouraging. A 1000-mile journey it is said begins with one step—start at the first 10%.

10% is not a burdensome quantity at any level. It is akin to the tithe in church circles, where the faithful are encouraged to give 10% of one's income to God's mission. Regardless of income level, parishioners give 10% and any additional offerings assist further to support the missions and upkeep of the church.

Look at the 10% in another way. As teenagers in my practice acquire part time jobs, I've often asked them "are you saving any of your paycheck, or do you spend it all as soon as you receive it?" Sometimes it's spent at the same store or mall that they work at. I then advise on the "pay yourself first" principle of saving 10% of each paycheck. That affords a small stash so you can treat yourself to something special occasionally and develop good saving habits to better serve in later working life.

Now that 10% is really ingrained, the point is that 10% is not painful, whether it is regarding weight loss, tithing, savings. It transcends many aspects of life, and the beauty in it is that the same principle works for everyone. If you can achieve greater than 10%, then that is profitable too. Just as you can tithe at any income level, even as a retiree, and you can teach children to tithe, and with more or reduced prosperity the numerical contribution changes, but the 10% remains the same proportion. Similarly, one can start a 10% weight reduction goal at any time and at any weight level.

Once your 10% goal is achieved and maintained, you reset 10% and slowly work toward the next target weight loss. There may be periods of plateau before the next weight loss is attained, but each increment of weight loss that is not regained, each dress size or pant size reduction should serve as encouragement to persevere. Remember, slow and steady wins the race as the saying goes. You're also developing habits for a lifetime, as one does with tithing and saving, which will serve for maintaining a steady state and be conducive to a healthier weight management regimen.

"The How To"

Weight loss programs are designed around methods of achieving the intake of fewer calories, whether you're skipping meals, leaving out food groups, counting calories or paying for pre-packaged meals. How then can you eat all the food groups, have the bread, and sample the desserts and lose weight? My mantra is "eat what you like but eat less of it" as in the United States particularly, it's the concept of portion sizes that need a major mental adjustment even given the constant availability of food. Skipping categories of foods can make you feel somehow deprived and there is no reason to be the "stick in the mud" at gatherings requesting no bread, no sugar, no fat, none of anything tasty, based on the diet program de jour that you've embarked on.

My advice is to decrease your current portion sizes by approximately 1/5 (one-fifth). That does not require working fractions or calculations, however, just take a little off everything on your plate or bowl.

Another way to look at it is, if you normally eat 5 slices of pizza, stop at 4 slices for a while. Once you get to not missing that 5th slice, cut to 3 slices. In time, you'll find that you're just fine with 2 or 3 slices. If you start with eating an entire pizza, then smile, you have some work to do, and should start ASAP. The focus is not specifically on fractions and actual calorie counts, but to decrease calories by reducing portion sizes. Remember, your satiety center is not in your belly, but in your brain. It's a reset of your mindset that must occur over time. The point is you can still enjoy pizza and your normal dietary repertoire, still be satisfied, enjoy the tastes that you have acquired, stop gaining weight and eventually lose and maintain it when you achieve your ideal weight. The fundamental principle of weight loss programs short of pills and injections and other unnatural methods is to reduce caloric intake. That's it! Root cause analysis, solution applied to the root cause.

Once you're cutting about 1/5 of your portion sizes for meals and snacks across the board, you're consuming fewer calories every day. Since you're still eating the foods that you like, or would normally eat, there is no depravation, no craving or feeling the need to cheat and "break diet", no need to hoard foods that you're pretending not to be allowed to eat because you're on whatever flavor of diet program. There is also no money spent, no "stick in the mud" attitude, no new schemes necessary. Just determination and conviction are required here.

You'll find that with time, you feel full on the smaller portions so that you can then adjust your portions further, until you wonder how you ate so much in the past before feeling satisfied as your satiety centers adjust gradually. You don't cut your portions in half or other large fractions that are hard to overcome, hence the projection of approximately 1/5. But over time, you find you may be eating half or even less of your original portion size and feeling full or at least satisfied.

If it takes prepackaged meals to reduce your portions then that's fine, however, it is not sustainable to order 3 meals per day and 2 snacks for prolonged periods of time or for a lifetime. You may need to use a smaller plate or bowl, estimate a palm or fist size or other visual aids, but you should be able to eyeball and reduce your portion sizes before you sit down to eat. Drink some extra water or juice (I always add water to my juices, as they are usually too sweet) if needed. It needs to become habitual to serve yourself less than you did previously. For snacks, eat one handful instead of a bag of cookies, chips etc., and for kids, it should be their handful, not the adult's, one less scoop of ice cream, one less or smaller slice of dessert, smaller portions of various desserts at one setting.

I hope that it goes without saying, that 2nd and 3rd portions should be rare and not an everyday affair where servings are concerned. Do cut out daily soda consumption, as it's said that one soda a day in addition to your normal intake can add about 20lbs to your weight in a year. Besides the empty calories in alcohol and soda get converted easily to fat, adding to your waistline as well as getting deposited in your liver, contributing to a fatty liver.

Do reduce your consumption of highly processed foods and too many foods containing high fructose corn syrup for the same reason as was just stated. Also, cut out too many after dinner snacks and consider that "if you eat it after dinner, you're wearing it".

Do make healthy choices in foods and snacks, add some fiber to the diet and other gut healthy foods to your repertoire. Get some healthy sustaining fuel for breakfast, as this is one of the most often skipped meals, and most people who are consistently gaining weight proudly state that they skip breakfast. It is important to get your day off to a good start with as little as a bagel and cheese and a small drink or a bowl of oatmeal and a tea or coffee, or other sustaining food combination that can fuel you to lunch.

I have been told too frequently, "we only eat healthy foods, we hardly eat out and don't eat fast food, so where is all this weight coming from? I don't understand". Then have you ever heard that too much of a good thing may be bad for you? Even fame and fortune, you just need to look around a bit to see that. There's where the concept of portion sizes and mindless eating and snacking also requires a mental shift, as vegetarians and people who eat "healthy foods" are often overweight and/or obese as well.

So, you can lose weight naturally, eat the foods that you generally like and not overhaul your entire way of eating and especially your sense of good taste. Sample the variety of food offered the world over, and it does not require spending sums of money or time. Adjust to eating lesser portions as it's the "too much that's bad for you".

> *"He who travels alone can start today, but he who travels with another must wait until the other is ready."*
> —Henry David Thoreau

CHAPTER 5

12 lbs. of Fudge/Doggy Bag It

You may have agreed with everything set forth so far but think that there are too many obstacles in your way. Habits are hard to break and take determination and consistency. It is stated that it takes about three weeks of working at it to change a habit. There is a myriad of excuses, and people and places to point fingers at that are all responsible for your continued weight gain, i.e., the "devil made me do it" concept.

I've literally had kids point to mom or dad and say she/he is to blame because that's who does the cooking. Mom makes too much; dad cooks large amounts of barbeque or roasts as if there's no such concept as leftovers and refrigerators. I often joke back, "but who's shoving it all down your gullet, eh?" Now there are the parents who shovel too much food onto kids' plates and insist that they must clean their loaded plates. That may have been a good attitude during the depression era, but not in times of abundance. I often admonish parents and grandparents not to encourage overeating, as this overcomes the child's natural biofeedback that regulates their satiety center and sets them up for lack of portion control later. I have at times recommended bringing grandma or dad in for a discussion on overfeeding kids or have them report back that "the doctor says", so that I could be the bad guy in facilitating the conversation.

I had a teenage patient, whom we'll call Julie, who was doing very well losing weight putting into practice the 10% goals and reducing portion sizes, although she could never get into the increasing activity part of our plan which will be covered in the next chapter. Julie plateaued sometimes but kept following up and progressing with reducing dress sizes. Her mom was generally supportive, but never could sign on to reducing the number of snacks in the cabinets or quantity of food that was made available. On one visit after Christmas, we had a follow-up appointment and I complemented her on not having gained weight through Thanksgiving and Christmas. I then asked, "how did you manage over the holidays?" She turned to her mother while relating that above all the usual offerings for the holidays, her mom made 12 lbs. of fudge for Christmas. The obvious question besides "who ate all of that fudge?" was, what did you do in that instance? Julie's response was, "I had a couple of pieces, but didn't eat it like I used to do". Congratulations, pats on the back, and hugs ensued. Eureka! Exactly the message that I'd been trying to impart. Enjoy some tasty food, no need to feel left out, sample everything and do not gain, possibly even lose weight.

There was a mother in one family who admitted that when she and her sisters emigrated as young adults and teens to the United States from Latin America, they were all slender then but now they were all overweight or obese. Her children though who were then pre-teens and teens were already overweight and on the march toward obesity. I have observed that trend over time even with moves from other West Indian islands to the US Virgin Islands (people hadn't even made it to the continental United States). Food was more plentiful and relatively cheap; the activity levels were significantly reduced, and the same trend as described for the family moving from Latin America to the United States was occurring with numerous families moving from the Caribbean to the US Virgin Islands. The realization must reset into a mindset of fuel up, enjoy, but don't overindulge.

Most restaurants in the United States serve portions that could suffice for 2 meals, particularly if you have the bread and appetizer and can't pass up on the scrumptious dessert menu. The exceptions are the expensive restaurants that serve large nicely decorated plates and small portions beautifully presented. For some, after barely affording 3 courses at a fancy restaurant, you feel like you could go through the fast-food drive through to fill up on the way home, except for spoiling the taste of the beautiful food you just had. For your regular restaurant fare though, the solution to enjoying all the courses and not gorging yourself is not the Romanesque Vomitorium, but "doggy-bag it". You get to taste the restaurant meal again and basically get 2 meals for the price of one. If everyone in the household brings home a doggy-bag, there's one less meal to prepare on the following day! That's a win-win situation right there and I'm saving you money instead of your spending money to get on my weight loss program. I've enjoyed the fresh bread and appetizer and soup so much that on numerous occasions I've had to doggy-bag my entire entre (sometimes I just take one bite to taste it freshly prepared). Restaurants will routinely bring out 4 or more spoons with one dessert. Plan to share the appetizers and desserts and enjoy all aspects of the meal.

"But it's an all you can eat buffet restaurant, now what"? By all means, sample everything that looks appealing to you. Save some room and get a sampling of the desserts too. However, if you're the kind who'll need to be rolled out in a barrel because you can hardly walk out, perhaps you don't want to do the buffet every Friday night eh. Live a little, don't overdo it.

I have seen people load up an obscene amount of butter on one piece of bread, so much so that I had to look away not to feel physically sickened. Why not savor the taste of butter on a nice piece of bread without excess. A sub sandwich is already substantially stuffed, so who needs a foot-long one as well as chips and a cookie.

We've all heard the one about a person ordering a large double or triple loaded burger, a supersized order of fries, a pastry, and a dessert and a "diet soda". The punch line being that the "diet soda" really offsets the three to four thousand calories that it's washing down.

Eat to live, but don't live to eat, says that you savor the flavor of life without the compulsion to overindulge.

So, "there are too many restaurants and fast-food joints in town", yes there are, sample some from time to time. I'm told, "Johnny doesn't eat much", but I'm observing Johnny moving by leaps and bounds off the weight chart. Means Johnny is eating more than he's burning for his level of activity consistently. "Janey only eats healthy foods because that's all I cook, none of that fast food stuff". Janey is consuming too much of a good thing then. Remember, it's the excess that hurts you. Vitamins are good for you, but excess of any vitamin, even if derived from juicing particular foods excessively and not from popping vitamin pills, can result in a medical diagnosis like Hypervitaminosis A, B or whichever one is being consumed in excess. Because it's "natural" doesn't mean it can't be harmful, keep that in mind also when embarking on dietary fads.

12 lbs. of fudge being available in addition to all the celebratory eating does not mean that you can't help but gain weight. It also doesn't mean that you crave what everyone else is eating and don't enjoy the foods offered for the season, the meal or get-together. Get to the Eureka moment where you can take some and leave some and let someone else enjoy some fudge.

Find your representation of the 12 lbs. of fudge that's tempting, magnetic, or that's just there, that causes you to overeat. How can you look at your 12lbs of fudge and have some, but like Julie, say "but I didn't eat it like I used to do". It may be that your primary portions are too large, or it's the second and third portions and dessert. For some people it's snacking all day, or after dinner and late-night snacks which you're wearing for sure, as there's no opportunity to burn those calories off. For some it's eating out of boredom or while distracted watching TV, playing video games, or even working. Perhaps you need to bypass certain isles at the supermarket and only venture down those isles now and then. Perhaps you don't go grocery shopping when you're hungry, so you're not tempted to purchase more food than you normally would. We can't close the fast-food stores, the supermarkets, and kitchens just so your 12 lbs. of fudge do not present a temptation. Figure out where and how you eat significantly more calories than you burn. Reprogram your satiety center to enjoy smaller portions, have no feelings of deprivation, have a happier and healthier body habitus. Enjoy 'happiness in a dish' like anyone else, anytime the situation arises.

"If you don't use it, you lose it."—*"A chair can Kill"*

CHAPTER 6

Sweat Equity

Now that you can easily take three meals a day, one or two snacks, occasionally indulge, and have stopped gaining weight, better still you're losing weight, would it hurt to move a muscle and burn some calories? It has been said that "a chair can kill", and prolonged sitting is now considered a risk factor not only for overweight and obesity, but for high blood pressure, heart disease, stroke, diabetes, and other health issues.

The sedentary lifestyle is fast becoming more critically so. We've gone from the main hinderance to moving having been the TV remote, to video games, then the computer (PC and laptop), to tablets, and now cell phones. Kids and adults alike are busy exercising the thumbs and index finger with very little activity for the rest of the body. Even at school, due to our risk averse society, there is reduced recess, and less playground activity permitted in the limited recess than was previously the norm.

I recall the two Christmas seasons when everyone made the excuse for spending hundreds of dollars on certain game consoles. The objective, as I was frequently told, was that it would help the kids and adults in the household to get much needed exercise and help with weight control. I thought then "yeah right, assuage your conscience that the hundreds of dollars are well spent on the high demand toy of the season". The game consoles all gathered dust and the kids and parents got no more exercise, while the weights kept going up.

It is sad that the ability to order everything online has decreased the necessity to stroll around a couple of stores to find a bargain. I get laughed at when I admit that I often find items online and then go to the store to make the purchase. Sometimes that backfired when I couldn't find the product in the store as advertised and had to return to purchase online. With home delivery for just about everything, even fast food can be delivered now. We can't even burn the few calories it takes to get into the car and go through the drive-thru to consume 3–4 thousand calories. Because we can, not because we must, and have delivery apps, let's order on our cell phone, have it delivered, and the girth goes on!

I recommend 20 to 30 minutes of exercise two to three times per week if you're trying to increase your usage of calories. Basically, do something to induce sweating. This also does not require any additional cost, as no gym membership is needed to get 20–30 minutes of "sweat equity". There is a variety of activities that will fit the bill. Weeding, gardening," brisk" walking, jogging if you're the jogging type as I must confess that jogging is not my thing, biking, swimming, or dancing to list a few. Find your thing or combination of activities that appeal to you.

My sweat exercise of choice which I do mostly on Saturday mornings, is what I call "Calypso-cise". I turn on my calypso music and dance and stretch. I have my mini carnival session, sweat, shower, and start the day. No set routine is necessary, or number of repetitions, just perpetual motion. You can just dance and incorporate sit-ups, push-ups, jumping jacks, lunges, abs, arms, legs, mix, and match working out different areas each session in between free dancing until you're tired and dripping with sweat. No two sessions are ever the same. Sometimes I add 1–2 lb. weights, resistance bands, or occasionally a hula-hoop, but the emphasis is to have fun and constant motion, even if it's just shuffling back and forth. I sometimes use other genres of music like disco, so you can make it Jazz-a-cise, salsa-cise, polka-cise, headbanger-cise, make it your free style. You don't require a lot of room either for my Sweat Equity-perpetual motion exercise routine. I do this mostly between the foot of my bed and the dresser. You need no more than a 2, 3, or 4-foot square area and some music to have an effective carnival like workout, sweat and get dog-tired. I call it my "4-square gym". The shower is then just a few steps away.

You can even do a few jumping jacks and stretches a few times a week while waiting for the shower to warm up from one day to another. If your job or school requires sitting all day, and then it's home to sit some more for the remainder of the day, then find reasons to get up and walk a bit at home and at work. Move a muscle or two throughout the day. While driving, occasionally suck in that gut, turn on some music and while at the stop light, use that time and move to the beat (don't get distracted on the road though or distract others). I sometimes try to move to music while cooking or even cleaning. It makes chores more profitable and possibly enjoyable.

A car does not get good value if it's in park or idle mode most of the time and doesn't get up even to city limit driving speeds. The engine and mechanisms need to be used from time to time. People have domesticated dogs and cats to the point where they get very little exercise and by and large have weight and mobility problems. People are now doing this to themselves. We need to get out of the house, "move a muscle", as delivery for everything should be a convenience or necessity, not a way of life, unless one is truly incapacitated. I once asked an elder doctor why I ran into him in the supermarket all the time. His reply was that he used it as a part of his exercise routine, as he walked around the perimeter of the store several times pushing his cart before he started to shop and walk between the isles. I've known of people who do a similar routine at the mall. In both instances, one can walk in airconditioned comfort and can do this regardless of the season of the year. I am not suggesting that we all do walk-a-thons in the grocery store, but there are many ways in which some regular exercise can be incorporated into otherwise mundane routines without significant cost or effort.

In nature, "if you don't use it, you lose it" and that applies to muscles, joints, and general fitness. You'll notice that after not using muscles for a while and then doing some exercise, whether gardening or working out, you wake up the next morning and find out where those muscles are that you just employed. Don't overdo it though, even if hurting because you hadn't used muscles for a while is normal. Hurting because you've damaged muscles and ligaments is a setback. My mantra applies here too, "moderation in all things won't hurt, it's the excess that hurts".

You may have to work up from sedentary to 20–30 minutes of cardio workout. I was told once, during a physical training test as an army physician (resident in training), that I did more of a walk than a run, but I was giving it all I had at the time, for not having trained and practiced. I had to train and retake the test. I found out too that sit-ups and push-ups are not as easy as they look. You may need to do modified sit-ups and push-ups at first or forever for that matter. Just use some muscles and joints here and there and as you lose weight you need to firm up too. It will pay dividends to your overall health and complement the healthy eating lifestyle that you've acquired.

"A body in motion stays in motion, a body at rest stays at rest"
—modification of Newton's 2nd Law of Motion.

"You can take the donkey to the water, but you cannot make him drink."

CHAPTER 7

Accountability

In numerous counseling sessions with kids and teens, whether it's for behavior (at home or school), bed wetting, and various situations, I've had to resort to saying " I can jump up and down and get exercised, so can your mom, teacher and whoever is interested in your fixing this issue, but if you do not decide to and make an effort, nothing can change". It's like the person who looks in the mirror and sees the obvious milk moustache, intends to wipe it off, but walks away neglecting to avoid the embarrassment of going around town until possibly the tenth person he encounters has the courage to point it out. It's funny isn't it, how we've all watched people with their fly down, tag hanging out of their clothes and debate whether we should be the one to embarrass them, as if it's not embarrassing enough for them to be going around not fixing the problem. Do "take a look" in the mirror and "act on what you see". The determination and the first step must be yours.

It took years of poor eating habits and sedentary lifestyle to get to a state of overweight, obesity, morbid obesity, and the changes that are made now need to develop into new habits for a lifetime going forward. Be rid of the crash diets and serial weight loss gimmicks. Afterall, "Rome wasn't built in a day".

You may have the courage and the tenacity to begin and maintain the process of looking at food differently entirely on your own and that's perfect. You may however find that it's necessary to partner with a friend or family member, a physician, or a weight management specialist, or group for a while. The accountability in reporting periodically, whether it be every two or three months and weigh-in, serves as to remind you to keep the focus on your goals, especially at times of plateauing and to give yourself a pat on the back for levels of success achieved. You're less likely to make excuses, find holidays every week to celebrate, and in other ways revert to your old ways of eating rather than establishing new habits.

You may only need to partner with some person or group for a short while, and that would be great. You may need a long-term partnership, and that's just as good. Know yourself, be true to yourself, and act accordingly to ensure that you are successful. Don't set yourself up for failure. You may live in a household or hang out with a group which makes the attempt to adjust your approach to eating as set forth here, feel like struggling against a strong headwind constantly. In this case, you need to partner for a long time with someone whose judgement you respect who can keep you accountable. Admit that it's sometimes challenging to reach great heights when the norm is to wade in the mire or in other words, to follow the path of least resistance. Please recall my 12 lbs. of fudge illustration, it's harder sometimes doing it alone and accountability can keep you focused until you develop self-propulsion.

I had a young adult patient chuckle as he stated" it's amazing that I can eat half of what I used to eat and still feel full". He also added that he'd occasionally eat a whole pizza in the past. He went on to talk about how in a few months he was already down a waist size and demonstrated how much less fat he could pinch at the belly than he did previously. After a pat on the back and thoroughly enjoying him revealing his success, I proceeded to show him his follow-up lab work as he beamed while calculating how many points his cholesterol and liver functions had improved. We parted with a plan to follow-up in 2 months for a weight check, so he'd remember to keep up the good work, while waiting at least 6 months to check lab work again.

Accountability is important too, because you'll inevitably hit a plateau after losing the first or second 10% of weight and you may feel like you're "stuck in the mud" for a while. That may be the key point at which you need someone to remind you of what you've accomplished and what your goals are. As new habits develop, hopefully they become second nature and then necessitate less need for handholding.

"Make hay while the sun shines."

"Never put off till tomorrow what you can do today."

CHAPTER 8

Medical Concepts Made Simple
Insulin Resistance and the Metabolic Syndrome

There are potentially serious health consequences to remaining overweight or obese. Overweight is considered a BMI (Body Mass Index) of above 25 and obese a BMI of 30 or above. These health problems relate to some of the following: easy fatigability, decreased mobility, joint pain especially in the knees and ankles, heart health, liver, kidneys and even skin, with ripples to other organ systems. The main health consequences that you may hear talked about are diabetes and the "metabolic syndrome". Factors contributing to the metabolic syndrome are explained here.

Insulin Resistance

Apart from constant, seemingly uncontrolled weight gain and persistent feeling of hunger, one outward sign of insulin resistance is dark discoloration of the skin on the neck as well as breast folds and folds in the arm pits. To most people, it looks like unwashed skin discoloration. This in medical circles is called Acanthosis Nigricans and if you check a fasting insulin level with this condition, it will be elevated. I've seen elevation as high as 191 in a child, while normal levels should be less than 20.

To back up though, you may ask what is insulin and why do I have a level? Insulin is a hormone that comes from an organ in the abdomen called the pancreas. It is released into the gut and blood to metabolize foods (carbohydrates, protein, and fat) and simply speaking, regulates the glucose or what we refer to as carbs in our blood and tissues. The pancreatic cells that make insulin release it into the blood stream when the glucose levels are high, that is after you have eaten, and decrease secretion when the glucose levels are low, that is when you have not eaten.

So, you eat a meal or a snack, and insulin jumps in to allow your body to process the food that you just ate or drank. Once the food is processed, the brain says, "that was good, I'm satisfied". Insulin flow shuts down, until the next meal or snack. The insulin level in your blood should rise in response to a meal but should return to baseline numbers between eating episodes and it's the in-between eating levels that your "fasting blood insulin level" lab work measures. The baseline insulin level is like the car in idle mode again, still working on glucose levels in your tissues, but not working hard. This is your biofeedback loop as God intended.

If you're frequently overeating, or grazing (snacking, drinking sodas, coffee, etc.,), that biofeedback loop gets short-circuited and your insulin production and shut down loop gets confused so to speak. Substituting diet soda and other low-calorie drinks and foods doesn't get you goody points either. My theory or way of explaining this is: as the load of empty calories hits your gut and blood stream and the 'insulin guys' are released; your brain gets mixed messages as they did not get to work on the number of calories they expected. These 'insulin guys' send messages back to the brain saying, "missing some calories here, where's the work?" Your brain responds, "eat some more as the 'insulin guys' are out in force, and they need material to work on". Subconsciously, your brain (Satiety center) and your pancreas are working against you. As the saying goes, you can't win, you can't break even, and what's worse, you can't even cop out". You literally feel hungry minutes after haven eaten so you feed the 'insulin guys' and the more that you graze and snack, the longer the insulin levels remain high. The more your insulin levels remain above normal, the hungrier you feel, and your brain thinks that it's being deprived of calories. Insulin is your friend, but it cannot be allowed to become your master. Your tissues get sensitized to the constant higher levels of circulating insulin and you develop "Insulin Resistance" of your tissues, so that your empty vs full feedback is damaged. Your body is now in this constant mode of packing away calories, mostly being converted to fat as it is persistently working as if you need to prepare for an oncoming famine and need to preserve a supply of energy that you might have to live off.

If you grew up going to what used to be called Sunday School, you've probably heard of the story of Joseph and the Pharaoh. Joseph successfully interpreted the Pharoah's disquieting dream, explaining that just ahead was 7 years of plenty (food and grain), followed by 7 years of famine. What needed to be done was to store as much provision during the seven years of plenty, so that the population could have enough rations to make it through the 7 years of no crops. Joseph got the job of organizing the storage and subsequent distribution of food and he saved the day.

Having insulin resistance is like being in a constant mode of needing to store away food for the coming famine, but it's mindless and totally driven by biochemistry. You literally feel hungry 10 to 20 minutes after a meal. If you live in the United States or anywhere that food is plentiful, whether you're rich or poor, when food is abundant, that famine is not coming; so, the fat stores never get used up or redistributed.

How do you break the cycle of Insulin Resistance and start the redistribution process? Let's look back at "root cause" and apply the solution to the root cause, which is where we started. My recommendation is to eat 3 scheduled meals a day of reasonable portions, stop frequent snacking/grazing and get that feedback loop between the brain and gut reestablished. Let the insulin levels operate as intended. If you can follow the advice laid out so far and reverse the bad biochemistry, you can stop gaining weight first, and then start on your 10% goals. As you reverse the process, it is amazing to see the fasting insulin levels decrease, as well as your HbA1C and fasting blood sugar levels, along with the weight.

Hemoglobin A1C (HbA1C)

This is a blood determination of the body's regulation of glucose(sugar) for the past 3-4 months. It is used to monitor how well diabetes is being controlled. At a level of 5.7 to 6.4, generally one is considered pre-diabetic. This is a good time to lose weight and try to reverse insulin resistance. Even in the diabetic range of HbA1C, above 6.4, lifestyle changes are important to avoid medication and the poor health aspects of diabetes.

Diabetes

Persisting Insulin Resistance will lead to increasing blood levels of glucose, which eventually leads to your pancreases "insulin guys" just not being effective and the persistent state of having elevated blood sugar levels is called Type 2 Diabetes. Not only does your blood glucose(sugar) remain high, even the urine has sugar that gets right through the kidneys, so you can check your fasting blood glucose for the level of diabetes or check the glucose in the urine. Type 2 Diabetes is what used to be called Adult-Onset Diabetes Mellitus but is now increasingly diagnosed in the pediatric population because of obesity.

In Type 1 Diabetes, or what used to be called Juvenile-Onset Diabetes Mellitus, the pancreas fails because of Auto-immune disease and the body does not put out insulin. That is why frequent insulin replacement injections, or an insulin pump is necessary to be able to eat and remain healthy. HbA1C is also used to monitor this type of diabetes. Our focus here is Type 2 Diabetes. The one that is associated with overweight and Insulin Resistance. If Type 2 diabetes is not reversed by lifestyle changes, there are medications that must be employed, and lack of control can eventually have significant health consequences. Those consequences can include poor healing of the skin, amputations (usually of the feet), kidney failure leading to dialysis, vision problems and heart disease. Diabetes also complicates treatment and healing from infections and other health problems.

"Everything in moderation won't hurt you, it's the excess that gets you."

CHAPTER 9

Medical Concepts Made Simple
Part 2

Fatty Liver

Here, we will focus on "Non-Alcoholic Fatty Liver". Recall in the discussion of Insulin Resistance, the liver as well as other undesirable areas of the body get to store fat deposits, as the main storage facility of excess calories is as fat, not as protein or starch. While fat deposits in other areas may look like a wider waistline, and signs of gaining weight, too much liver tissue taken over by fat deposits destroys the good liver tissue and the liver cannot do its work properly, and inflammation occurs which can lead to liver disease. Signs of the liver not functioning properly can be seen in blood tests, Aspartate Aminotransferase (AST) and Alanine Transaminase (ALT), which are used to assess liver health. The more elevated those values, the worse the condition of the liver. Fatty liver infiltration may lead to cirrhosis (inflammation) and liver cancer.

Cholesterol Levels

The combination of insulin resistance, Hypertension (high blood pressure), abdominal fat and cholesterol abnormalities sets an individual up for what is referred to as the "Metabolic Syndrome". This syndrome puts one at risk for cardiovascular disease as well as Type 2 Diabetes. Your cholesterol profile is to some extent inherited. It can be modified by lifestyle, to include diet and exercise and weight reduction.

A cholesterol profile test or lipid profile test measures the levels of fat in the blood. Usually, your doctor will discuss HDL (High Density Lipoprotein) which is referred to as the good cholesterol, and Total cholesterol, LDL (Low Density Lipoprotein) and Triglycerides, which are referred to as the bad cholesterols.

The HDL cholesterol is believed to be protective against cardiovascular disease especially if it is above 70 and the ratio of HDL compared to the bad cholesterols, Total, LDL and Triglycerides is important in cardiovascular risk. Basically, the higher your HDL the better for you and the higher the total, LDL and Triglycerides, the worse your risk.

To illustrate, picture the cholesterol issue this way. Having too much bad cholesterol is like having a major intersection crowded by a massive number of people who are spilling out from the roads onto the sidewalk and adjoining square in a downtown area.

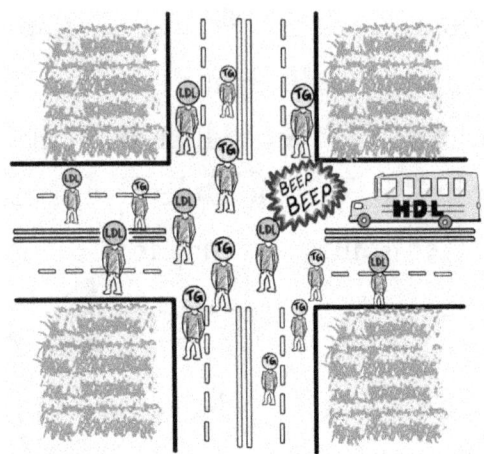

Bad cholesterol clogs blood vessels

One way to clear out the obstruction while all those people remain downtown is to get a fleet of buses and cars and move those people into a neat line of parked vehicles. You've effectively removed the clog. Picture the HDL as the vehicles that managed the clog. It would be nice also if some of the crowd left the scene, which would be like lowering your cholesterol level. Either way, you can now move pedestrians and unrelated vehicles through the formally clogged downtown, which represents your arteries and veins.

Weight reduction, exercise, more fiber in the diet, less carbohydrates and processed simple sugary foods will all help to reverse a poor cholesterol profile/ratio. Triglycerides, which are important in the Metabolic Syndrome, are responsive to dietary changes. If all else fails a doctor may need to prescribe medication to assist with cholesterol management, but whatever can be done without medication is best done that way as all medications have side effects.

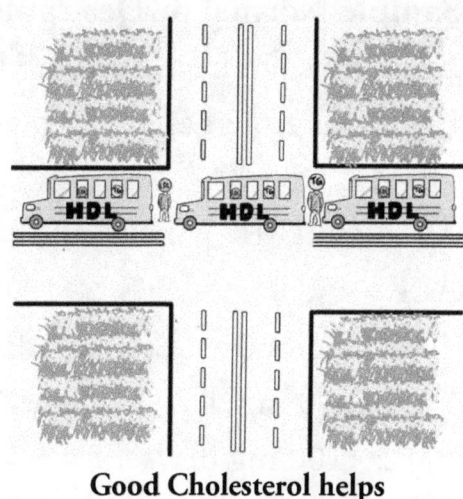

Good Cholesterol helps clear blood vessels

Inflammation

Excess weight causes inflammatory changes in your body. Inflammation can be evident in a common lab value in your blood work called the ESR (Erythrocyte Sedimentation Rate). The ESR is an indirect or non-specific indication of inflammation and will be elevated for any reason that there is sustained inflammation. It is common to see elevated ESR values in obese individuals. There are hidden areas of inflammation as previously mentioned in the liver, as well as other tissues due to obesity, but there are visible areas of inflammation such as hip, knee and ankle pain and discomfort from carrying excess weight.

Hopefully the explanations of the medical terminology will facilitate dialogue with your physician or dietary management personnel.

Sample Normal or Desirable LAB VALUE Numbers

Fasting Insulin Level: <20 mlU/mL
Fasting Glucose Level: <99 mg/dL
HbA1C: <5.6%
AST: <30 U/L
ALT: <45 U/L
Total Cholesterol: <200 mg/dL
HDL: >60 mg/dL
LDL: <100 mg/dL
Triglyceride: <100 mg/dL
ESR: <20 mm/hr

Keep in mind that laboratories and medical centers will have slightly different ranges of normal lab values, therefore, consider overall desirable or target lab values.

"Repetition is good for the human brain."

CHAPTER 10

New Habits and Recap

Here are some useful tips to cement healthy lifestyle changes. Healthy eating habits once established should serve for a lifetime of eating well and eating in proper proportions for growth, maintenance, or weight reduction.

- ❖ Eat at a designated place and time. Most of the excess calories are consumed at home, just as most accidents are said to occur at home. Sit at the table for meals and most snacks. This eliminates eating in front of the TV, computer, videogames, and other activities, as countless calories are consumed mindlessly while otherwise distracted. Much of this consumption is unnecessary, at least not for fuel or for dispelling hunger. If you can't bother to stop and sit at the table, you probably do not need to eat then and there and can spare those calories. That can be one strategy to draw attention to how excessive calories are being eaten.

- ❖ Eat as much as possible as a family or household. That lends itself to better meal preparation, more well thought out and likely more balanced meals. It also allows for interaction, conversation about school, work, issues, serving as a time-out, and for greater bonding. Life can get very busy, especially with kids at home, extracurricular activities, projects, and work schedules. Ritualized eating assists with improved quality of life.

❖ Incorporate fiber and healthy foods into your dietary routine. It will pay dividends regarding your cholesterol, heart health and bowel health. I often find myself asking "do you sample a vegetable once in a while?" as the vegetable food group is usually the one lacking in a dietary survey. It starts with toddlers as veggies are always the first food group to fall off the preferred list. I see significantly more iron, vitamin B12, and folic acid deficiencies in recent years, especially among teens and young adults whose food choices do not allow for a balance of nutrients. Do eat a green leafy vegetable occasionally. No one seems to eat liver or beets anymore. I mention liver and even the moms do the eye roll or grimace. As for beets, you're probably wondering what a beet is! Feel free to look it up. There are many ways to make one pot meals and perhaps blend in the vegetables so that they do not stand out. There are frozen vegetable packs that steam up in minutes and instant oatmeal, grits or cream of wheat that take no time to prepare compared to dry cereals. There is no need to skip meals for lack of time, or consistently eat highly processed foods that turn into fat quickly. Between breakfast, lunch, and dinner, one could surely incorporate all the food groups at least over a couple of days.

❖ If you cannot get all the food groups well represented at least every couple of days, the vitamin deficiencies can be avoided by taking a multivitamin supplement. There is no added load of calories in taking a multivitamin. Ensure that it is complete and adds iron, calcium, and folate. Remember though, that vitamins, minerals, and trace elements are only needed in small amounts, and like anything else, too much must be eliminated or stored by the body. The extra work on the excretory and storage systems of the body can be harmful at some level and "too much of a good thing" is in poor taste. If a little is good for you, more is not necessarily better, and you run into problems from taking too much of any specific vitamin, leading to diagnoses like Hypervitaminosis A, B or whatever you take in excess. Unless you have a measured deficiency of a particular vitamin or mineral, it's best to take a multivitamin and limit the quantity of any one supplement. Everything should be done in moderation.

- ❖ Skip the center isles of the supermarket sometimes. That is where a lot of the snacks and processed foods reside. If the house is not stocked with the temptation to snack constantly, or the opportunity to sneak or otherwise overeat, it's less likely to become habitual, and being truly hungry by mealtime is a good thing. Let that insulin level drop to fasting levels by mealtime. Keeping the desserts and snacks in good proportions, or as occasional treats won't upset the proverbial apple cart.

Recap

The underlying issue is not that you have specifically eaten too much fat to begin with, or that you ate some bread and carbs, or that you already eat healthy foods anyway. Rice and bread are staples in the diet in much of the world where obesity is not a problem. I recall one day at university, there was rice porridge for breakfast and white rice for lunch and dinner in the cafeteria at my residence hall and my remarking 'what's with the white rice all day, at least some seasoned rice for lunch or dinner would be more appealing'. The issue is eating too much period, compared to your level of activity. The excess calories are turned into fat by your own body and stored. You go on a starvation diet of whatever variety, and by the time you fit into that bridesmaid dress or suit and pat yourself on the back, you're on the way to refilling those fat cells. The reason is you haven't acquired a new approach to food that is sustainable. Besides, while you're in starvation mode, the last thing that your body will burn off for fuel is fat.

You can stop gaining and gradually lose weight without buying into a program, without avoiding entire food groups or purchasing prepackaged meals. If you feel you need to do those activities as well, by all means, "be all that you can be", but do address the root cause and apply the solution to the cause. You can eat a balanced diet, participate fully in events and celebrations involving food, and work toward a desirable weight and improved overall health.

- ❖ Recognize that persistent weight gain occurs because you constantly eat far more calories than you are burning. Begin a process of gradual reduction of portion sizes and adjust your satiety center.
- ❖ Eat 3 meals per day and one or two snacks. Allow for fasting insulin levels to return to baseline levels between meals. Incorporate a balanced diet with moderation as the steering principle. It's the excess that hurts. Portion sizes, Portion sizes! My common advice is "eat what you like, just eat less of it," that way you have no cravings for things that can't be on your diet program. Adjust your portion size down slowly by comfortable increments.
- ❖ Decrease consumption of highly processed foods and of soda, whether diet or regular variety.
- ❖ Aim to reduce your current weight by 10% over a reasonable time and adjust your goals so that you build on your successes.
- ❖ Get active, move a little, sweat regularly. Exercise helps to burn calories and is good for one's general health and wellbeing.
- ❖ Get started. Determination, perseverance, and accountability are of paramount importance, especially if you are surrounded by household members who regularly overeat and are not signed on to your new purpose. Encourage someone to embark on this path with you. You do not have to trudge along alone. At least find someone who can coach or monitor your progress and occasionally give you a pat on the back.

❖ Acquire a different mindset about food and eating. Reestablish good biochemistry and biofeedback.

Lose and maintain weight as nature intended, naturally. Work toward the "Eureka!" moment when you can look at 12 lbs. of fudge, be content to savor some, but not feel the compulsion to gorge yourself. Eating can be a pleasure as well as serving as fuel. You only live once, as the saying goes. You may indulge on Thanksgiving, birthdays, Christmas, Easter, and other events of significance in your life or culture. You can't eat that way regularly or eat mindlessly. Have some cheesecake, eat some bread, fresh bread is delightful even with nothing spread on it. Eat to live, for sustenance and enjoyment. Bon Appetit!

Sample weight charting graph.

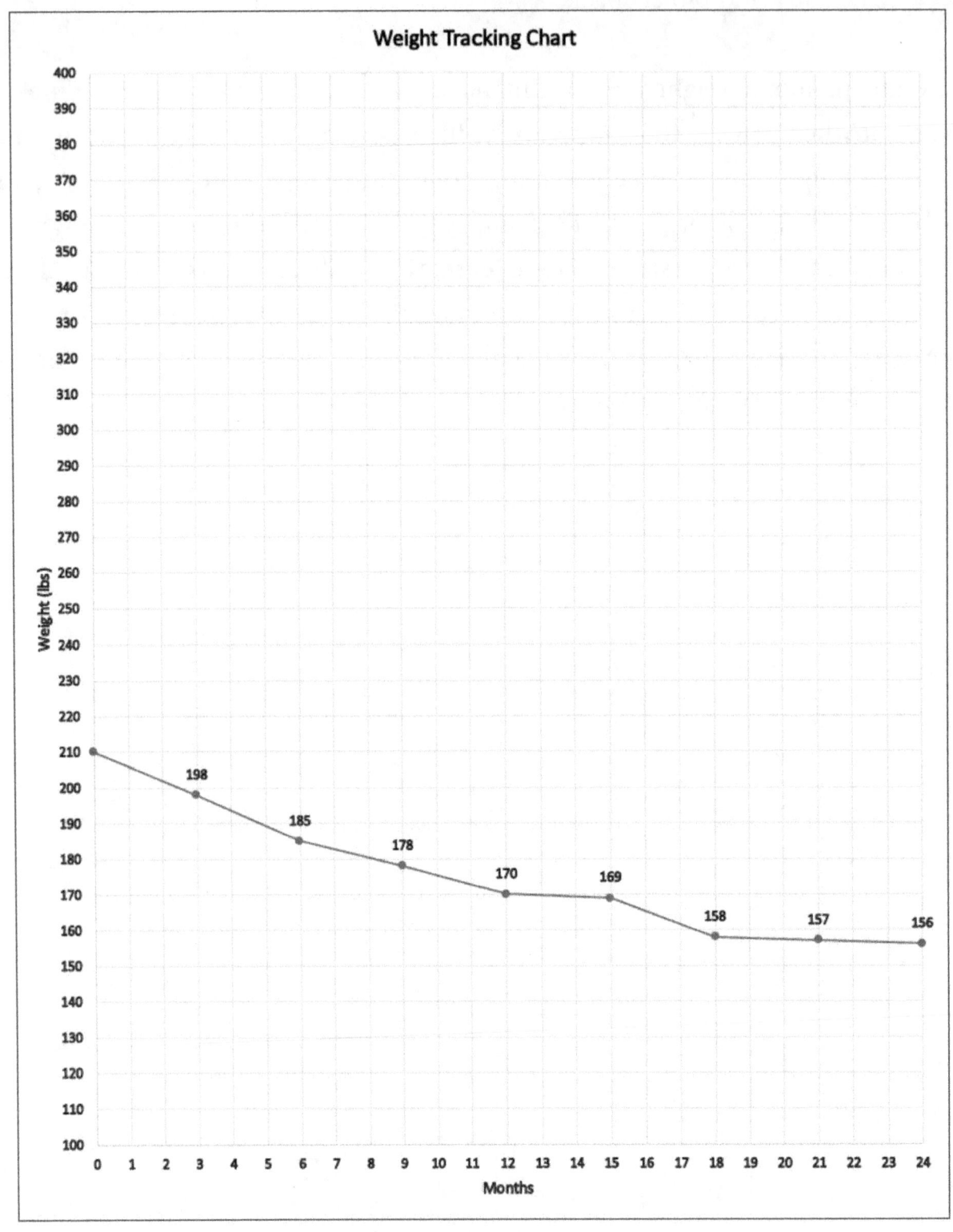

Chart your own weight progress in pounds (lbs) for 1 year.

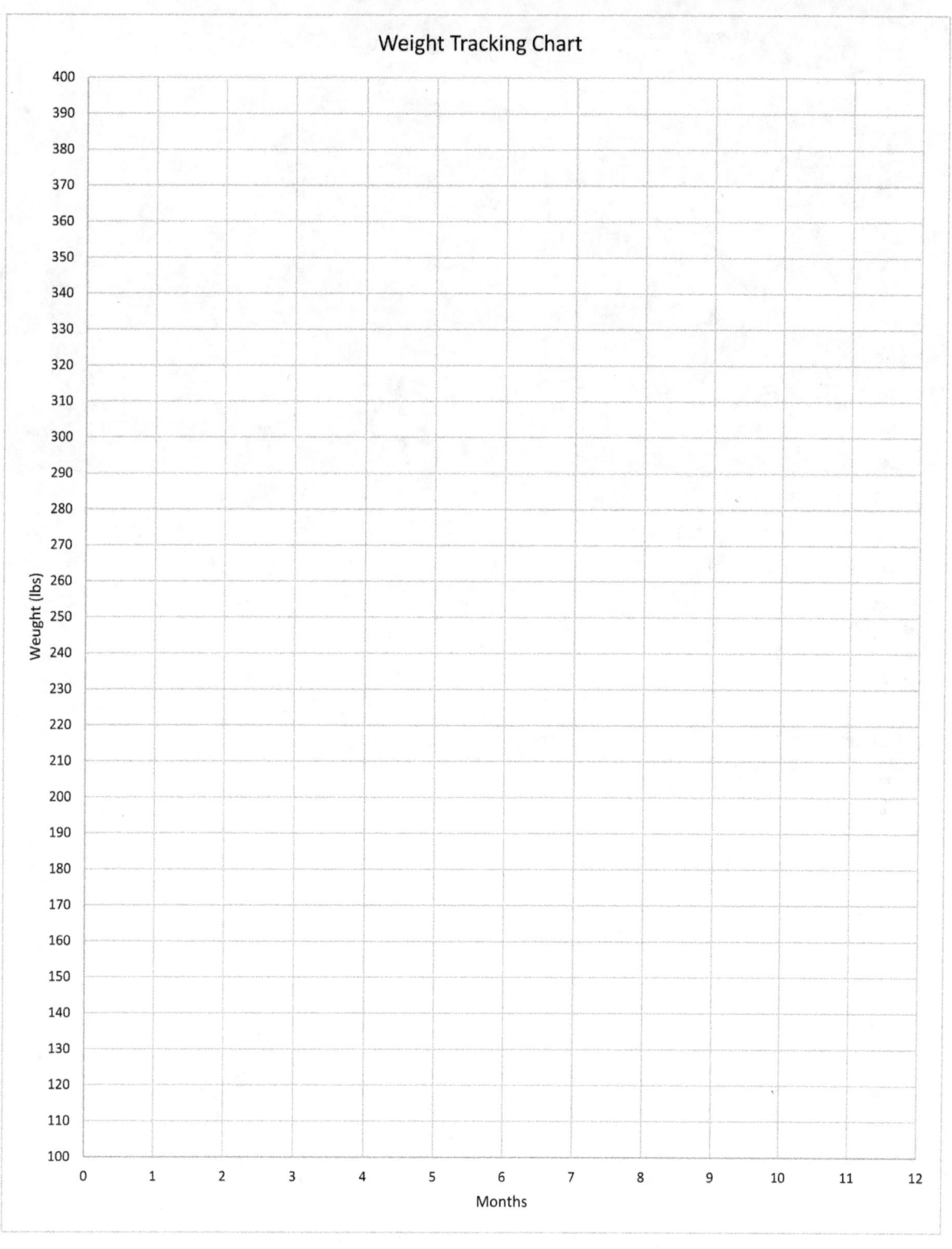

Chart your own weight progress in Kilograms (Kg) for 1 year.

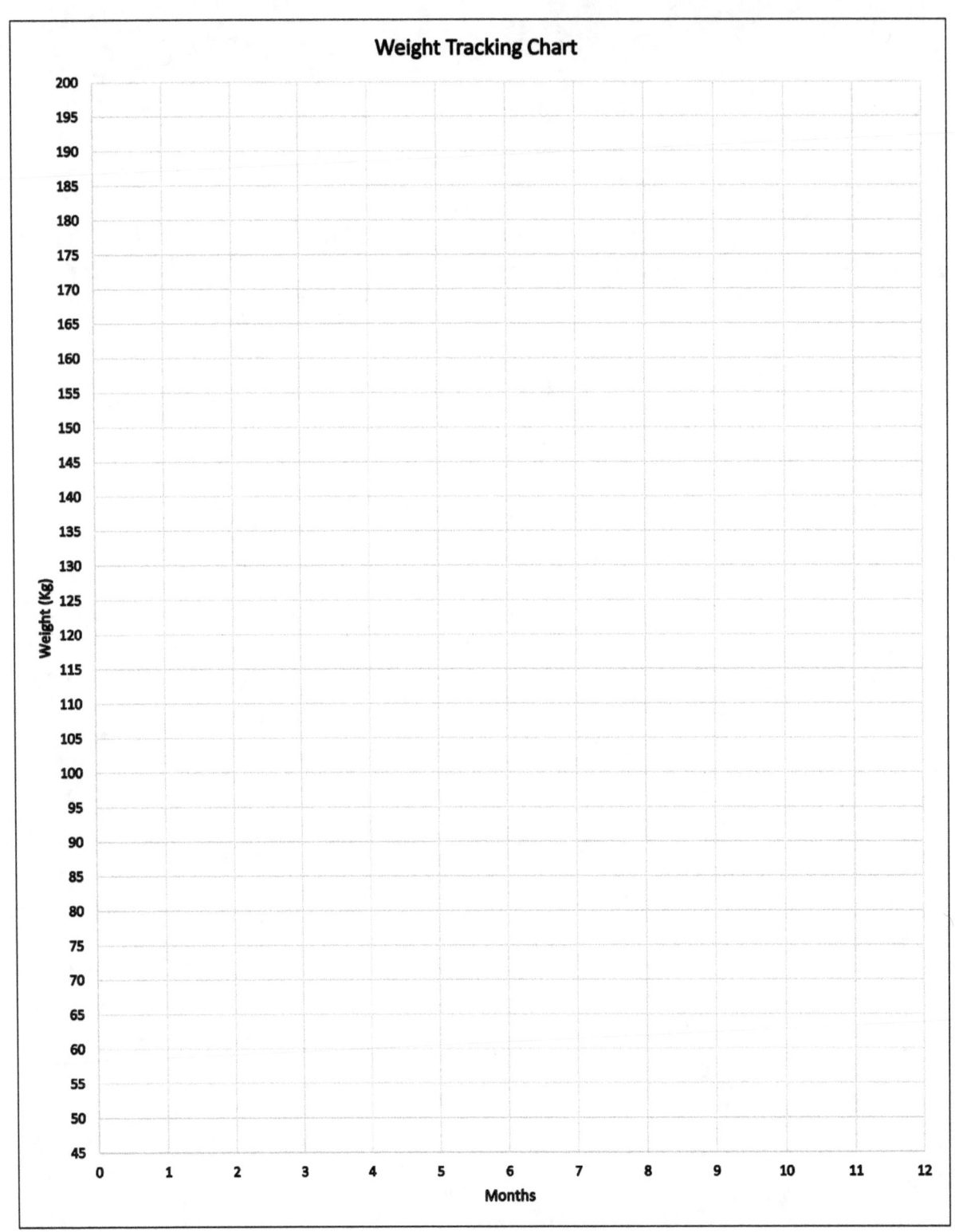

Chart your own weight progress in pounds (lbs) for 2 years.

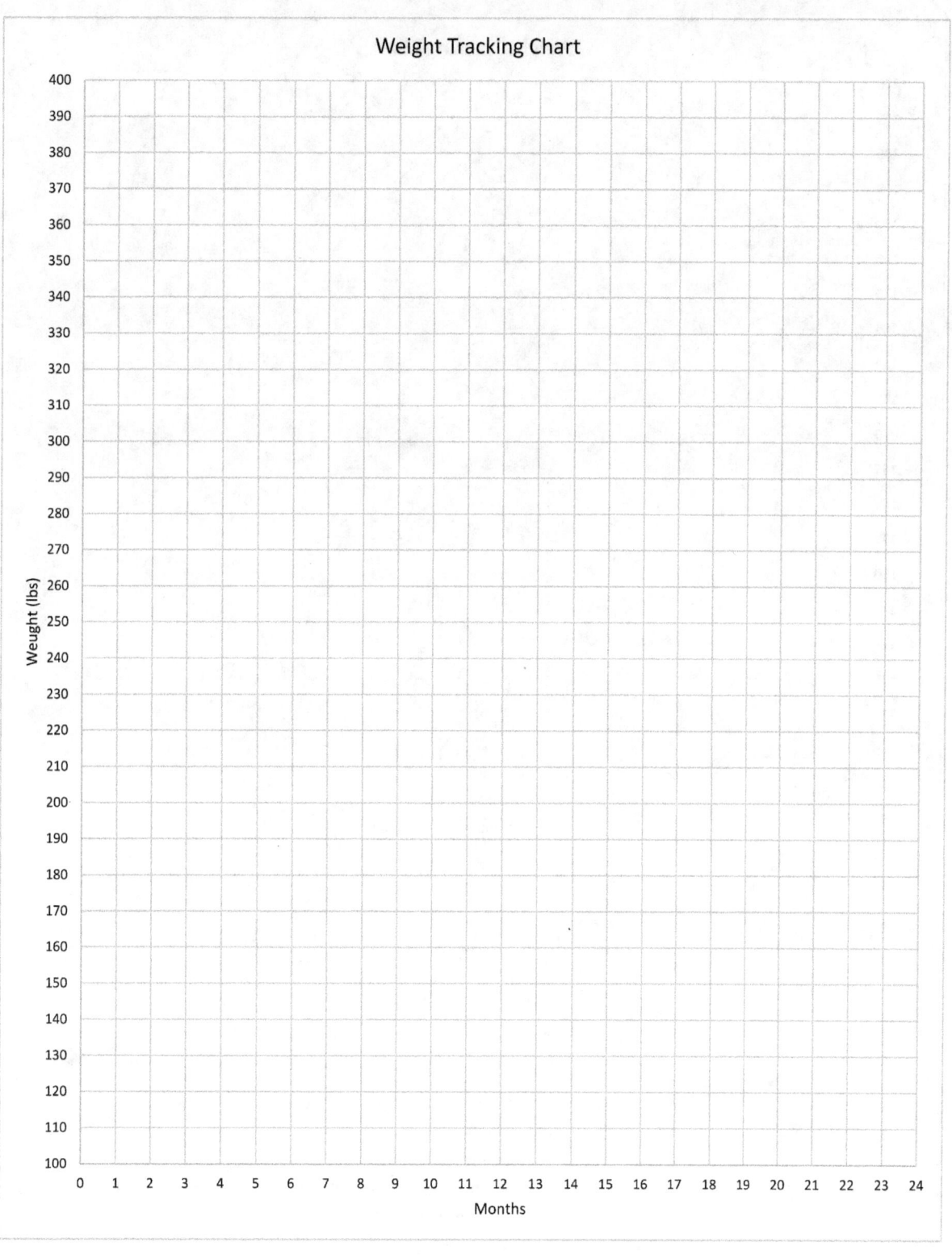

Chart your own weight progress in Kilograms (Kg) for 2 years.

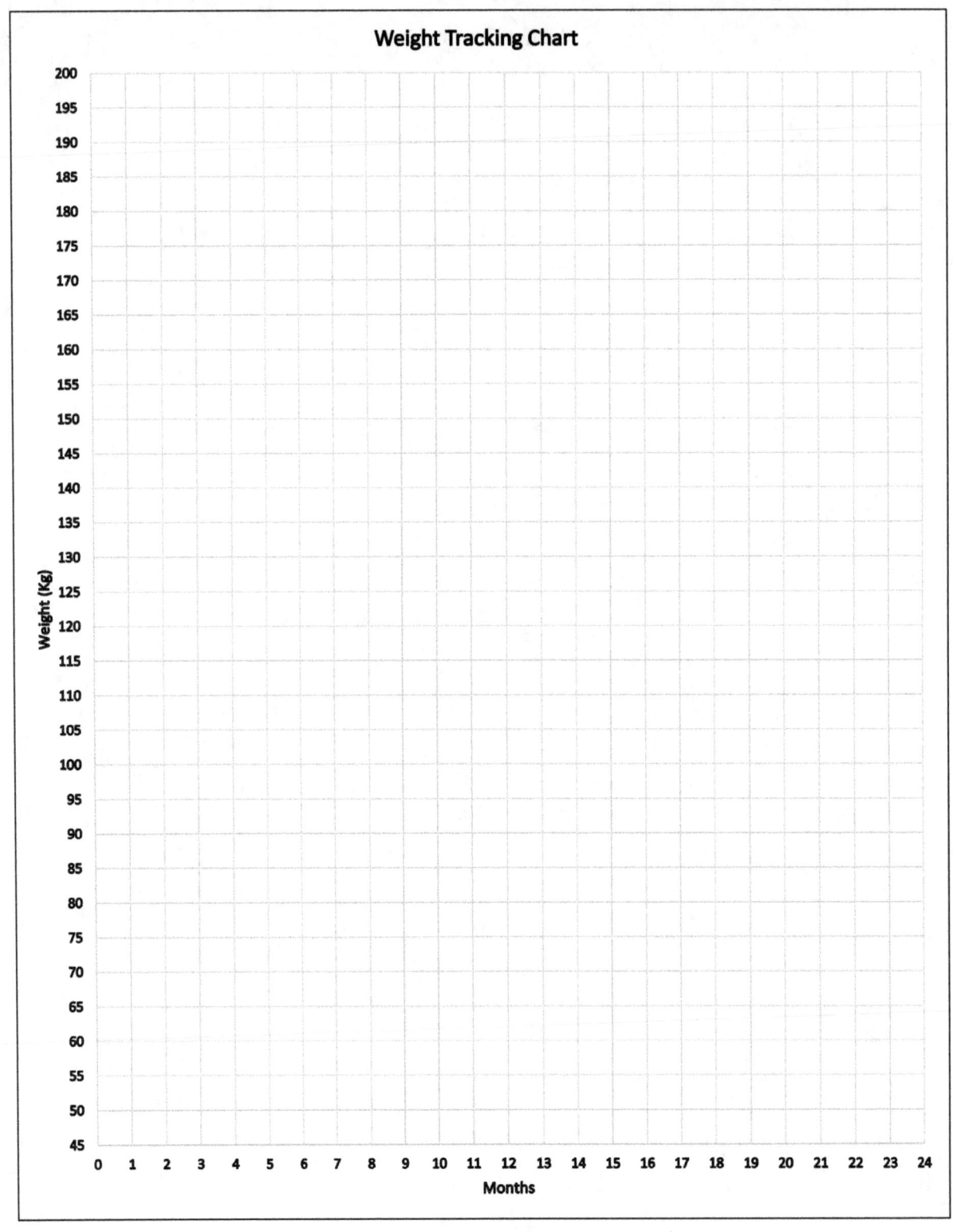

www.ingramcontent.com/pod-product-compliance
Lightning Source LLC
LaVergne TN
LVHW081454060526
838201LV00050BA/1794